Family Keto Diet Dessert Cookbook

The Best Recipes Collection for Healthy and Tasty Dessert

Jodi D. Ryan

Sommario

Introduction

Are you seeking a simple way to cook well balanced meals in the comfort of your very own house? Are you searching for simple kitchen tools that will help you prepare some abundant and tasty dishes for you and also your loved ones? Well, if that holds true, then this is the most effective overview you could use. This cooking guide offers to you the best and also most ingenious cooking tool readily available nowadays. We're talking about the immediate pot This initial and also helpful pot has gained numerous followers all over the globe as a result of the reality that it's so easy to use and since it can assist you cook numerous tasty meals. You can prepare easy morning meals, lunch recipes, treats, appetizers, side dishes, fish as well as seafood, meat, chicken, vegetable and treat dishes immediate pot. This brings us to the 2nd part of this guide. This journal concentrates on using the immediate pot to make the very best Ketogenic dishes. The Ketogenic diet regimen is much more than a straightforward fat burning program. It's a way of living that will boost your health and wellness as well as the method you look. This low-carb and high-fat diet will certainly get your body to a state of ketosis. The diet regimen assistance you create even more ketones as well as for that reason it will certainly enhance your metabolic process as well as your power degrees.

The Ketogenic diet will show its several advantages in an issue of minutes as well as it will certainly help you look far better.

Ketogenic Instant Pot Dessert Recipes

Plums and Berries Compote

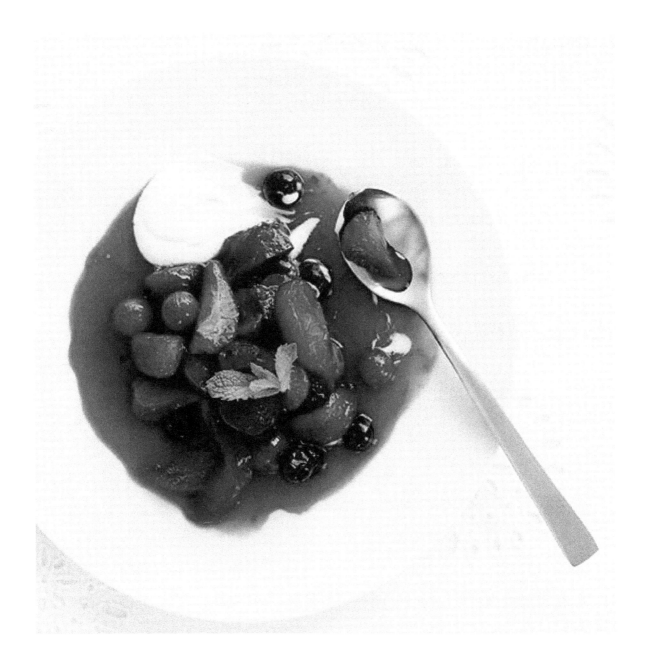

Preparation time: 10 minutes

Cooking time: 20 minutes

Servings: 4

Ingredients:

- 1 cup plums, pitted and halved

- 1 cup blueberries

- 2 tablespoons lemon juice

- 1 and ½ cups water

- ¾ cup swerve

- 1 teaspoon vanilla extract

Directions:

In your instant pot, mix the plums with the berries and the rest of the ingredients, put the lid on and cook on High for 20 minutes. Release the pressure naturally for 10 minutes, divide the compote into bowls and serve.

Nutrition: calories 43, fat 1.2, fiber 0.1, carbs 1, protein 0.5

Keto Vanilla Crescent Cookies

Preparation time: 15 minutes

Cooking time: 19 minutes

Servings: 7

Ingredients:

- 1/3 cup butter, softened

- 3 oz almond flour

- 1.5 oz almonds, grinded

- 2 ½ tablespoons stevia

- ½ teaspoon vanilla extract

- 1 tablespoon Erythritol

- 1 cup water, for cooking

Directions:

Knead the dough from almond flour, butter, almonds, stevia, and vanilla extract. Then roll the dough into the log shape and cut into 7 pieces. Make the shape of crescents. Pour water and insert the trivet in the instant pot. Line the trivet with baking paper and place the crescents on it. Cook the crescent cookies in the manual (high pressure) for 19 minutes. When the time is finished, make a quick pressure release. Sprinkle every crescent cookie in Erythritol.

Nutrition: calories 182, fat 17.8, fiber 2.1, carbs 3.9, protein 3.9

Lime Watermelon Compote

Preparation time: 5 minutes

Cooking time: 10 minutes

Servings: 4

Ingredients:

- 1 and ½ cups watermelon, peeled and cubed

- 2 tablespoons lime juice

- 2 cups water

- 3 tablespoons swerve

Directions:

In your instant pot, mix the watermelon with the rest of the ingredients, put the lid on and cook on High for 10 minutes.

Release the pressure fast for 5 minutes, divide the mix into bowls and serve really cold.

Nutrition: calories 40, fat 1, fiber 0.1, carbs 0.2, protein 0.6

Vanilla Muffins

Preparation time: 10 minutes

Cooking time: 15 minutes

Servings: 4

Ingredients:

- 4 tablespoons almond flour

- 1 tablespoon cream cheese

- 1 egg, beaten

- 1 teaspoon vanilla extract

- ¼ teaspoon baking powder

- ¼ teaspoon apple cider vinegar

- 4 teaspoons Erythritol

- 1 cup water, for cooking

Directions:

In the bowl combine together cream cheese, egg, vanilla extract, baking powder, apple cider vinegar, and Erythritol. When the mass is homogenous, add almond flour and stir until smooth. Pour water and insert the trivet in the instant pot. Fill the muffin molds with muffins batter and transfer on the trivet. Close the lid and cook the dessert on manual (high pressure) for 15 minutes. When the time is finished, make a quick pressure release and remove the muffins from the instant pot immediately.

Nutrition: calories 188, fat 16, fiber 3, carbs 6.4, protein 7.6

Heavy Cream and Raspberries Ramekins

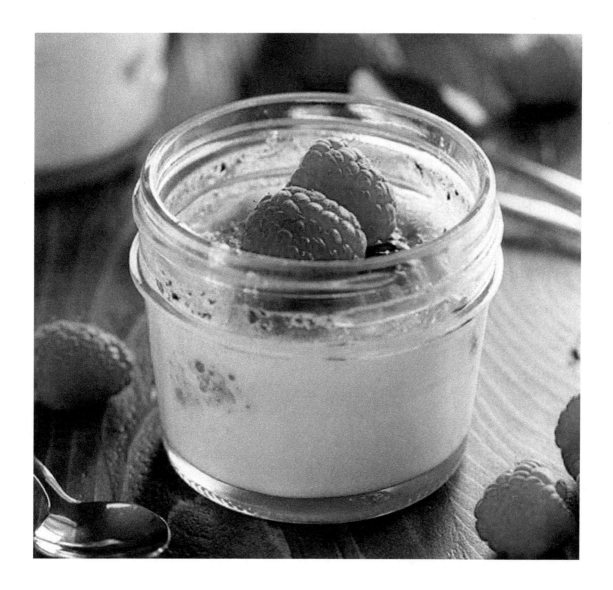

Preparation time: 5 minutes

Cooking time: 8 minutes

Servings: 4

Ingredients:

- 2 cups raspberries

- 1 cup heavy cream

- ¼ cup swerve

- 2 tablespoons ghee, melted

- 1 teaspoon vanilla extract

- ½ teaspoon ginger powder

- 1 cup water

Directions:

In a bowl, mix the raspberries with the cream and the rest of the ingredients except the water, whisk and divide into ramekins. Put the water in the instant pot, add the steamer basket, put the ramekins inside, put the lid on and cook on High for 8 minutes. Release the pressure fast for 5 minutes, and serve cold.

Nutrition: calories 195, fat 17.9, fiber 4, carbs 7.5, protein 1.4

Fat Bomb Jars

Preparation time: 8 minutes

Cooking time: 6 minutes

Servings: 4

Ingredients:

- 1 tablespoon coconut oil

- 1 pouch sugar-free chocolate chips

- ½ cup whipped cream

- 3 tablespoons almond butter

- ¼ teaspoon ground cardamom

Directions:

Toss the coconut oil in the instant pot and melt it on sauté mode. After this, add ground cardamom and chocolate chips. Melt the mixture and switch off the instant pot. After this, transfer the chocolate mixture into the bowl. Add whipped cream and almond butter. Stir the mixture until smooth and homogenous. With the help of the scooper place the mixture into the glass jars.

Nutrition: calories 172, fat 15.6, fiber 1.5, carbs 7, protein 3.1

Coconut Pecans Cream

Preparation time: 10 minutes

Cooking time: 15 minutes

Servings: 4

Ingredients:

- 1 cup pecans, chopped

- 1 cup coconut cream

- ½ cup coconut, unsweetened and shredded

- 4 tablespoons swerve

- 1 teaspoon vanilla extract

- 1 cup water

Directions:

In a bowl, mix the pecans with the rest of the ingredients except the water, whisk and divide into ramekins. Put the water in the instant pot, add the steamer basket inside, add the ramekins, put the lid on and cook on High for 15 minutes. Release the pressure naturally for 10 minutes and serve cold.

Nutrition: calories 176, fat 17.6, fiber 2.2, carbs 5, protein 1.7

Blueberry Clusters

Preparation time: 10 minutes

Cooking time: 6 minutes

Servings: 6

Ingredients:

- 1.5 oz dark chocolate

- 1 tablespoon coconut oil

- 1/3 cup blueberries

Directions:

Toss coconut oil in the instant pot. Set sauté mode for 6 minutes and melt the oil. Add dark chocolate and stir well. Cook the mixture until it is homogenous. After this, line the baking tray with baking paper and arrange the blueberries on it into 6 circles. Then sprinkle every "blueberry circles" with melted chocolate mixture and let dry. Store the cooked clusters in the glass jar with the closed lid up to 2 days.

Nutrition: calories 67, fat 5.3, fiber 1.2, carbs 7.9, protein 0.6

Chocolate and Brazil Nuts Bread

Preparation time: 10 minutes

Cooking time: 30 minutes

Servings: 4

Ingredients:

- 1 cup coconut milk

- 2 eggs, whisked

- 2 teaspoons vanilla extract

- 1 cup swerve

- 1 cup brazil nuts, peeled and chopped

- 2 cups coconut flour

- 2 ounces chocolate, melted

- ¼ teaspoon baking powder

- 2 cups water

- Cooking spray

Directions:

In a bowl, combine the coconut milk with the eggs and the rest of the ingredients except the cooking spray and the water and whisk well. Grease a loaf pan with the cooking spray and pour the bread mix inside. Add the water to the instant pot, add the steamer basket, put the loaf pan inside, put the lid on and cook on High for 30 minutes. Release the pressure naturally for 10 minutes, cool the bread down and serve.

Nutrition: calories 253, fat 19.7, fiber 1.8, carbs 6.8, protein 5.2

Strawberry Cubes

Preparation time: 10 minutes

Cooking time: 7 minutes

Servings: 4

Ingredients:

- 4 strawberries

- 1 tablespoon heavy cream

- 1 teaspoon butter

- 1 tablespoon cocoa powder

Directions:

Put the strawberries in the freezer for 5-10 minutes. Preheat the instant pot bowl on sauté mode for 3 minutes. Then add butter and melt it. Add heavy cream and cocoa powder. Whisk the mixture until smooth and turn off the instant pot. After this, let the chocolate mixture cool to room temperature. Dip every strawberry in the chocolate mixture and let to dry it for 3-4 minutes.

Nutrition: calories 28, fat 2.6, fiber 0.6, carbs 1.8, protein 0.4

Greek Pudding

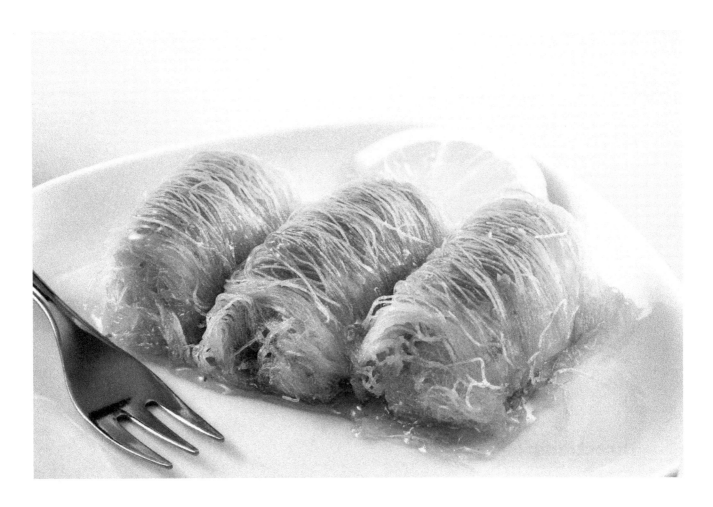

Preparation time: 10 minutes

Cooking time: 30 minutes

Servings: 4

Ingredients:

- 1 and ½ cups coconut flour

- 1 teaspoon baking powder

- ½ teaspoon vanilla extract

- 2 eggs, whisked

- 2 cups Greek yogurt

- ½ cup swerve

- 3 tablespoons coconut flakes

- 2 cups water

Directions:

In a bowl, mix the flour with the baking powder and the rest of the ingredients except the water, whisk well and pour into a pudding pan. Add the water to the instant pot, add the steamer basket, put the pudding pan inside, put the lid on and cook on High for 30 minutes. Release the pressure naturally for 10 minutes and serve the pudding cold.

Nutrition: calories 94, fat 4.3, fiber 0.4, carbs 1.5, protein 4.9

Avocado Brownies

Preparation time: 15 minutes

Cooking time: 14 minutes

Servings: 12

Ingredients:

- 1 avocado, peeled, pitted

- 1 tablespoon cocoa powder

- 1 tablespoon almond butter

- 1 teaspoon vanilla extract

- 1 egg, beaten

- 4 tablespoons almond flour

- ½ teaspoon baking powder

- 3 tablespoons Erythritol

- ½ teaspoon apple cider vinegar

- 1 cup water, for cooking

Directions:

Churn the avocado till the creamy texture. Add cocoa powder, almond butter, vanilla extract, and egg. Mix up the mixture until it is smooth. Then add almond flour, baking powder, Erythritol, and apple cider vinegar. Stir the mass well and pour in the instant pot baking mold. Flatten the surface and cover it with the foil. Pierce the foil with the help of the toothpick. Pour water and insert the trivet in the instant pot. Place the baking mold with a brownie on the trivet and close the lid. Cook the dessert for 14 minutes on manual mode (high pressure). When the time is finished, make a quick pressure release and remove the brownie. Discard the foil and cut the brownie into bars.

Nutrition: calories 103, fat 9.1, fiber 3, carbs 2.4, protein 3.1

Pecans and Plums Bread

Preparation time: 10 minutes

Cooking time: 30 minutes

Servings: 4

Ingredients:

- 1 cup coconut flour

- 3 eggs, whisked

- 1 tablespoon vanilla extract

- 1 and ½ cups swerve

- 2 cups plums, pitted and chopped

- 2 cups coconut milk

- 2 tablespoons pecans, chopped

- ¼ teaspoon baking powder

- 2 cups water

- Cooking spray

Directions:

In a bowl, combine the coconut flour with the eggs and the rest of the ingredients except the cooking spray and the water and whisk well. Grease a loaf pan with the cooking spray and pour the bread mix inside. Add the water to the instant pot, add the steamer basket, put the loaf pan inside, put the lid on and cook on High for 30 minutes. Release the pressure naturally for 10 minutes, cool the bread down, slice and serve.

Nutrition: calories 348, fat 23.5, fiber 3.1, carbs 6.6, protein 7.2

Cheesecake Bites

Preparation time: 15 minutes

Cooking time: 12 minutes

Servings: 2

Ingredients:

- 2 teaspoons cream cheese

- ¼ teaspoon vanilla extract

- 2 tablespoons peanut flour

- ¼ teaspoon coconut oil

- 1 egg, beaten

- 1 teaspoon Splenda

- 1 cup water, for cooking

Directions:

In the mixing bowl mix up cream cheese with vanilla extract, peanut flour, coconut oil, egg, and Splenda. When the mixture is smooth, transfer it in the muffin molds. Pour water and insert the trivet in the instant pot. Place the muffin molds on the trivet and close the lid. Cook the cheesecake bites on manual mode (high pressure) for 12 minutes. When the time is over, allow the natural pressure release for 10 minutes.

Nutrition: calories 76, fat 4.7, fiber 0.6, carbs 3.5, protein 4.3

Chocolate Cheesecake

Preparation time: 10 minutes

Cooking time: 40 minutes

Servings: 6

Ingredients:

- 2 tablespoons ghee, melted

- 1 cup heavy cream

- 2 ounces chocolate, melted

- ½ cup swerve

- 12 ounces cream cheese, soft

- 1 and ½ teaspoon vanilla extract

- 2 eggs, whisked

- Cooking spray

- 1 cup water

Directions:

Grease a spring form pan with cooking spray and leave it aside. In a bowl, mix the ghee with the chocolate, the cream and the rest of the ingredients except the water, whisk well and pour into the pan. Add the water to the instant pot, add the steamer basket, put the pan inside, put the lid on and cook on Low for 40 minutes. Release the pressure naturally for 10 minutes, and serve the cheesecake cold.

Nutrition: calories 282, fat 25.4, fiber 0.2, carbs 5.8, protein 5.5

Coconut Crack Bars

Preparation time: 10 minutes

Cooking time: 8 minutes

Servings: 4

Ingredients:

- 1 cup unsweetened coconut flakes

- 4 tablespoons coconut oil

- 1 egg, beaten

- 2 tablespoons coconut flour

- 2 tablespoons monk fruit

Directions:

In the mixing bowl combine together 3 tablespoons of coconut oil, coconut flour, egg, and coconut flakes. Then add monk fruit and stir the mixture well with the help of the spoon. The prepared mixture should be homogenous. After this, toss the remaining coconut oil in the instant pot and heat it up on sauté mode. Meanwhile, make the small bars from the coconut mixture. Place them in the hot coconut oil in one layer and cook for 1 minute from each side. Dry the cooked coconut bars with a paper towel if needed.

Nutrition: calories 218, fat 21.2, fiber 3.3, carbs 6.1, protein 2.9

Plums and Rice Pudding

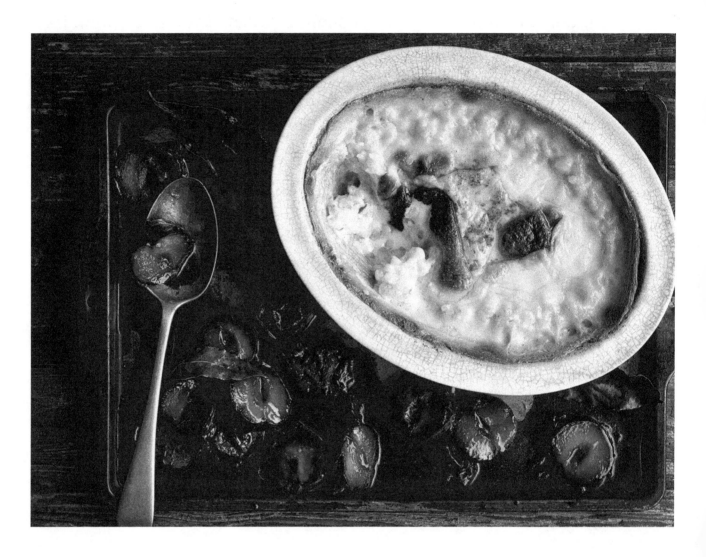

Preparation time: 6 minutes

Cooking time: 20 minutes

Servings: 4

Ingredients:

- 2 cups coconut milk

- 1 cup cauliflower rice

- ½ cup plums, pitted and chopped

- ¼ cup heavy cream

- 2 eggs, whisked

- ½ cup swerve

- ½ teaspoon vanilla extract

Directions:

In your instant pot, mix the cauliflower rice with the plums and the rest of the ingredients, put the lid on and cook on High for 20 minutes. Release the pressure fast for 6 minutes, divide the pudding into bowls and serve cold.

Nutrition: calories 339, fat 27.7, fiber 2.7, carbs 6.5, protein 5.7

Keto Blondies

Preparation time: 15 minutes

Cooking time: 30 minutes

Servings: 4

Ingredients:

- 2 oz almond flour

- 2 oz coconut flour

- ½ teaspoon baking powder

- 3 tablespoons Erythritol

- 1 egg, beaten

- 2 tablespoons almond butter, softened

- 1 teaspoon walnuts, chopped

- 1 cup water, for cooking

Directions:

Line the instant pot baking tray with baking paper. After this, in the mixing bowl combine together almond flour, coconut flour, baking powder, and Erythritol. Add egg, almond butter, and walnuts, With the help of the spoon stir the mass until homogenous. Then transfer it in the prepared baking tray and flatten well the surface of the dough. Pour water in the instant pot and insert the trivet. Place the tray on the trivet and close the lid. Cook the blondies for 30 minutes on manual mode (high pressure). When the time is over, make a quick pressure release. Cool the blondies to the room temperature and cut into serving bars.

Nutrition: calories 180, fat 14, fiber 4.9, carbs 9, protein 7.3

Cinnamon Berries Custard

Preparation time: 10 minutes

Cooking time: 15 minutes

Servings: 4

Ingredients:

- 3 eggs, whisked

- 2 cups coconut milk

- 1/3 cup swerve

- 1 tablespoon ghee, melted

- ½ cup heavy cream

- 1 tablespoon cinnamon powder

- ½ cup raspberries

- 1 teaspoon vanilla extract

- 1 and ½ cups water

Directions:

In a bowl, combine the eggs with the milk and the rest of the ingredients except the water, whisk well and transfer to a pan that fits the instant pot. Add the water to the instant pot, add the steamer basket, put the pan inside, put the lid on and cook on High for 15 minutes. Release the pressure naturally for 10 minutes, divide the mix in bowls and serve really cold.

Nutrition: calories 1276, fat 26.7, fiber 2.4, carbs 6.2, protein 4.9

Low Carb Nutella

Preparation time: 10 minutes

Cooking time: 5 minutes

Servings: 4

Ingredients:

- 3 oz hazelnuts

- 2 tablespoons coconut oil

- 1 teaspoon of cocoa powder

- 1 teaspoon Erythritol

- 2 tablespoons heavy cream

Directions:

Place coconut oil in the instant pot. Set sauté mode and heat it up for 3-4 minutes until the oil is melted. Then add Erythritol and cocoa powder. Whisk it well until homogenous. After this, add heavy cream. Stir the mixture until smooth and switch off the instant pot. After this, grind the hazelnuts. Add melted coconut oil mixture to the grinded hazelnuts. Stir well with the help of the spoon. Store Nutella in the fridge for up to 5 days.

Nutrition: calories 219, fat 22.6, fiber 2.2, carbs 4, protein 3.4

Ginger and Cardamom Plums Mix

Preparation time: 10 minutes

Cooking time: 15 minutes

Servings: 4

Ingredients:

- 3 cups plums, pitted and halved

- 2 cups heavy cream

- 1 tablespoon ginger, grated

- 3 tablespoons swerve

- 2 teaspoons vanilla extract

- ¼ teaspoon cardamom, ground

Directions:

In your instant pot, combine the plums with the cream and the rest of the ingredients, put the lid on and cook on High for 15 minutes. Release the pressure naturally for 10 minutes, divide the mix into bowls and serve cold.

Nutrition: calories 241, fat 22.4, fiber 0.9, carbs 6, protein 1.7

Cheesecake Fat Bombs

Preparation time: 20 minutes

Cooking time: 30 minutes

Servings: 2

Ingredients:

- 1 egg yolk

- 2 tablespoons cream cheese

- 1 teaspoon swerve

- ¼ teaspoon vanilla extract

- 3 tablespoons heavy cream

- 1 teaspoon coconut flakes

Directions:

Whisk the egg yolk with swerve until smooth. Then add heavy cream and pour the liquid in the instant pot. Stir it until homogenous and cook on manual mode (low pressure) for 30 minutes. Meanwhile, mix up together cream cheese with vanilla extract, and coconut flakes. When the time is over and the egg yolk mixture is cooked, open the instant pot lid. Combine together cream cheese mixture with egg yolk mixture and stir until homogenous. Place the mixture in the silicone muffin molds and transfer in the freezer for 20 minutes. The cooked cheesecake fat bombs should be tender but not liquid.

Nutrition: calories 146, fat 14.4, fiber 0.1, carbs 2.4, protein 2.6

Chocolate Cake

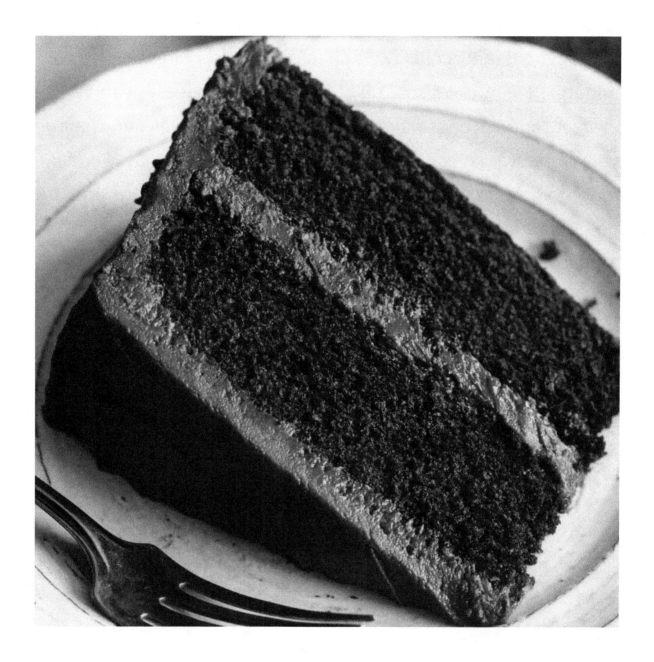

Preparation time: 10 minutes

Cooking time: 30 minutes

Servings: 4

Ingredients:

- 1 and ½ cups almond flour

- 1 cup cocoa powder

- Cooking spray

- 1 cup coconut flour

- 2 teaspoons baking powder

- 2 teaspoons baking soda

- ¼ cup flaxseed meal

- ½ cup ghee, melted

- 1 cup swerve

- 4 eggs, whisked

- 1 cup almond milk

- 1 teaspoon vanilla extract

- 2 cups water

Directions:

In a bowl, combine the almond flour with the cocoa, coconut flour and the rest of the ingredients except the cooking spray and the water and whisk really well. Grease a cake pan with the cooking spray and pour the cake mix inside. Add the water to the instant pot, put the steamer basket, add the cake pan inside, put the lid on and cook on High for 30 minutes. Release the pressure naturally for 10 minutes, cool the cake down, slice and serve.

Nutrition: calories 344, fat 33.1, fiber 3.4, carbs 5.8, protein 8.1

Peanut Butter Balls

Preparation time: 10 minutes

Cooking time: 5 minutes

Servings: 2

Ingredients:

- •1 tablespoon peanuts

- •1 tablespoon butter

- •1 teaspoon Erythritol

- •4 tablespoons coconut flakes

Directions:

Set sauté mode on your instant pot for 5 minutes. Place the butter inside and melt it. Meanwhile, finely chop the peanuts. Add them in the melted butter. After this, add Erythritol and coconut flakes. Stir the mixture until homogenous. With the help of the scooper make 2 balls and chill them in the fridge.

Nutrition: calories 112, fat 11.4, fiber 1.3, carbs 2.3, protein 1.6

Chocolate Cookies

Preparation time: 10 minutes

Cooking time: 30 minutes

Servings: 4

Ingredients:

- 2 eggs, whisked

- ½ cup ghee, melted

- 2 tablespoons heavy cream

- 2 teaspoons vanilla extract

- 2 and ¾ cups almond flour

- ¼ cup swerve

- 1 cup chocolate chips

- Cooking spray

- 1 and ½ cups water

Directions:

In a bowl, mix the eggs with the ghee and the rest of the ingredients except the cooking spray and the water and whisk well. Put the water in the instant pot, add the steamer basket inside, arrange the cookies inside, spray them with cooking spray, put the lid on and cook on High for 30 minutes. Release the pressure naturally for 10 minutes, and serve the cookies cold.

Nutrition: calories 257, fat 21.4, fiber 0.7, carbs 12.5, protein 3.1

Cinnamon Muffins

Preparation time: 10 minutes

Cooking time: 18 minutes

Servings: 4

Ingredients:

- 4 teaspoons cream cheese

- 1 teaspoon ground cinnamon

- 1 tablespoon butter, softened

- 1 egg, beaten

- 4 teaspoons almond flour

- ½ teaspoon baking powder

- 1 teaspoon lemon juice

- 2 scoops stevia

- ¼ teaspoon vanilla extract

- 1 cup of water, for cooking

Directions:

In the big bowl make the muffins batter: mix up together cream cheese, ground cinnamon, butter, egg, almond flour, baking powder, lemon juice, stevia, and vanilla extract. When the mixture is smooth and thick, pour it into the 4 muffin molds. Then pour the water in the instant pot and insert the trivet. Place the muffins on the trivet and close the lid. Cook them for 18 minutes on Manual mode (high pressure). When the time is over, make a quick pressure release and cool the cooked muffins well.

Nutrition: calories 216, fat 19.2, fiber 3.3, carbs 7, protein 7.7

Coffee Cake

Preparation time: 10 minutes

Cooking time: 40 minutes

Servings: 4

Ingredients:

- 1/3 cup brewed coffee

- 1 and ½ cups almond flour

- ½ cup ghee, melted

- 1 and ½ cups swerve

- ½ teaspoon baking powder

- 4 eggs, whisked

- 1 teaspoon vanilla extract

- Cooking spray

- 1 cup water

Directions:

In a bowl, combine the coffee with the flour and the rest of the ingredients except the cooking spray and the water and whisk well. Grease a cake pan with the cooking spray and pour the cake mix inside. Put the water in the instant pot, add the steamer basket, put the cake pan inside, put the lid on and cook on High for 40 minutes. Release the pressure naturally for 10 minutes, cool the cake down, slice and serve.

Nutrition: calories 195, fat 20, fiber 0, carbs 0.5, protein 3.8

Keto Fudge

Preparation time: 10 minutes

Cooking time: 6 minutes

Servings: 5

Ingredients:

- ¾ cup of cocoa powder

- 1 oz dark chocolate

- 4 tablespoons butter

- 1 tablespoon ricotta cheese

- ¼ teaspoon vanilla extract

Directions:

Preheat the instant pot on sauté mode for 3 minutes. Place chocolate in the instant pot. Add butter and ricotta cheese. Then add vanilla extract and cook the ingredients until you get liquid mixture. Then add cocoa powder and whisk it to avoid the lumps. Line the glass mold with baking paper and pour the hot liquid mixture inside. Flatten it gently. Refrigerate it until solid. Then cut/crack the cooked fudge into the serving pieces.

Nutrition: calories 155, fat 13.8, fiber 4.6, carbs 10.7, protein 3.3

Nutmeg Pudding

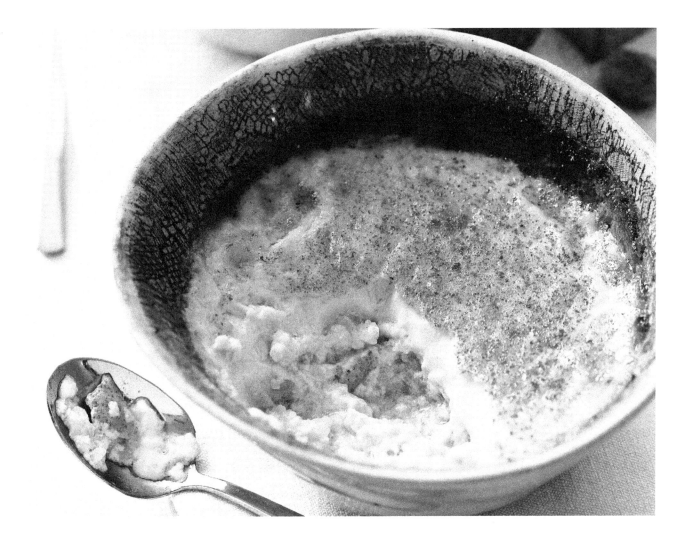

Preparation time: 10 minutes

Cooking time: 30 minutes

Servings: 6

Ingredients:

- 2 cups water

- Cooking spray

- ½ cup swerve

- 4 eggs, whisked

- 1 cup heavy cream

- ½ cup almond flour

- 1 teaspoon nutmeg, ground

- ½ teaspoon baking soda

- 2/3 cup ghee, melted

Directions:

In a bowl, mix the swerve with the eggs and the rest of the ingredients except the cooking spray and the water and whisk. Grease a pudding pan with the cooking spray and pour the pudding mix inside._Put the water in the instant pot, add the steamer basket, put the pudding pan inside, put the lid on and cook on High for 30 minutes. Release the pressure naturally for 10 minutes, cool the pudding down and serve.

Nutrition: calories 235, fat 24.7, fiber 0.1, carbs 0.7, protein 3.2

Fluffy Donuts

Preparation time: 20 minutes

Cooking time: 14 minutes

Servings: 2

Ingredients:

- 1 tablespoon organic almond milk

- 1 egg, beaten

- ¼ teaspoon baking powder

- ¼ teaspoon apple cider vinegar

- 1 teaspoon ghee, melted

- 1 teaspoon vanilla extract

- 1 tablespoon Erythritol

- ¾ teaspoon xanthan gum

- 1 teaspoon flax meal

- 1 scoop stevia

- ¼ teaspoon ground nutmeg

- 1 tablespoon almond flour

- 1 cup water, for cooking

Directions:

Make the dough for the donut: in the big bowl mix up almond milk, egg, baking powder, apple cider vinegar, ghee, vanilla extract, Erythritol, xanthan gum, flax meal, and almond flour. With the help of the spoon stir the mixture gently. Then knead the non-sticky dough. Cut it into small pieces and put it in the silicone donut molds. Pour water and insert the trivet in the instant pot. Place the silicone molds with donuts on the trivet and close the lid. Cook the donuts on manual mode "high pressure" for 14 minutes. When the time is over, make a quick pressure release and open the lid. In the shallow bowl mix up together ground nutmeg and stevia. Sprinkle every donut with the stevia mixture.

Nutrition: calories 233, fat 18.9, fiber 5.4, carbs 9.3, protein 9.1

Chocolate Chips Balls

Preparation time: 5 minutes

Cooking time: 6 minutes

Servings: 6

Ingredients:

- 1 cup chocolate chips

- 2 tablespoons ghee, melted

- 2/3 cup heavy cream

- 2 tablespoons swerve

- ¼ teaspoon vanilla extract

- 1 cup water

Directions:

In a bowl, combine the chocolate chips with the ghee and the rest of the ingredients except the water, stir well and shape medium balls out of this mix. Put the water in the instant pot, add the steamer basket, put the balls inside, put the lid on and cook on High for 6 minutes. Release the pressure fast for 5 minutes and serve the chocolate balls cold.

Nutrition: calories 350, fat 23.8, fiber 1.4, carbs 6.9, protein 3.6

Coconut Muffins

Preparation time: 15 minutes

Cooking time: 12 minutes

Servings: 6

Ingredients:

- ½ cup coconut flour

- 2 eggs, beaten

- ¼ cup Splenda

- ½ teaspoon vanilla extract

- 3 teaspoons coconut flakes

- ¼ cup heavy cream

- 1 teaspoon baking powder

- 1 teaspoon lemon zest, grated

●1 cup water, for cooking

Directions:

Make the muffins batter: In the bowl whisk together coconut flour, eggs Splenda, vanilla extract, coconut flour, heavy cream, baking powder, and lemon zest. Use the hand blender to make the batter smooth. Then pour water in the instant pot and insert the trivet. Pour muffins batter in the muffin molds. Then transfer the molds on the trivet and close the lid. Cook the desert on manual mode (high pressure) for 12 minutes. When the time is over, allow the natural pressure release for 5 minutes.

Nutrition: calories 48, fat 3.8, fiber 0.7, carbs 1.9, protein 2.2

Coconut and Cocoa Doughnuts

Preparation time: 10 minutes

Cooking time: 20 minutes

Servings: 4

Ingredients:

- ¼ cup swerve

- ¼ cup flaxseed meal

- ¾ cup coconut flour

- 1 teaspoon baking powder

- 1 teaspoon vanilla extract

- 2 eggs, whisked

- 3 tablespoons ghee, melted

- ¼ cup coconut milk

- 1 tablespoon cocoa powder

- Cooking spray

- 1 cup water

Directions:

In a bowl, mix the swerve with the flaxmeal and the rest of the ingredients except the cooking spray and the water and stir well. Grease a doughnut pan with the cooking spray and divide the mix. Add the water to the instant pot, add the steamer basket, put the pan inside, put the lid on and cook on High for 20 minutes. Release the pressure naturally for 10 minutes, cool the doughnuts down and serve.

Nutrition: calories 196, fat 17.3, fiber 2.7, carbs 4.5, protein 4.7

Raspberry Pie

Preparation time: 15 minutes

Cooking time: 25 minutes

Servings: 6

Ingredients:

- ¼ cup raspberries

- 1 tablespoon Erythritol

- 3 tablespoons butter, softened

- ¼ teaspoon baking powder

- ½ cup almond flour

- 1 tablespoon flax meal

- 1 teaspoon ghee, melted

- 1 cup water, for cooking

Directions:

Blend raspberries with Erythritol in the blender until smooth. Then in the mixing bowl combine together butter, baking powder, almond flour, flax meal, and knead the dough. Cut it into 2 pieces. Then put one piece of dough in the freezer. Meanwhile, roll up the remaining piece of dough in the shape of a circle. Grease the instant pot baking mold with ghee. Place the dough circle in the prepared baking mold. Then pour the blended raspberry mixture over it. Flatten it with the help of the spoon. Then grate the frozen piece of dough over the raspberries. Pour water and insert the trivet in the instant pot. Cover the pie with foil and put it on the trivet. Close the lid and cook the pie on manual mode (high pressure) for 25 minutes. When the time is finished, make a quick pressure release. Discard the foil from the pie and let it cool to the room temperature.

Nutrition: calories 118, fat 11.6, fiber 1.7, carbs 3, protein 2.4

Chocolate Balls

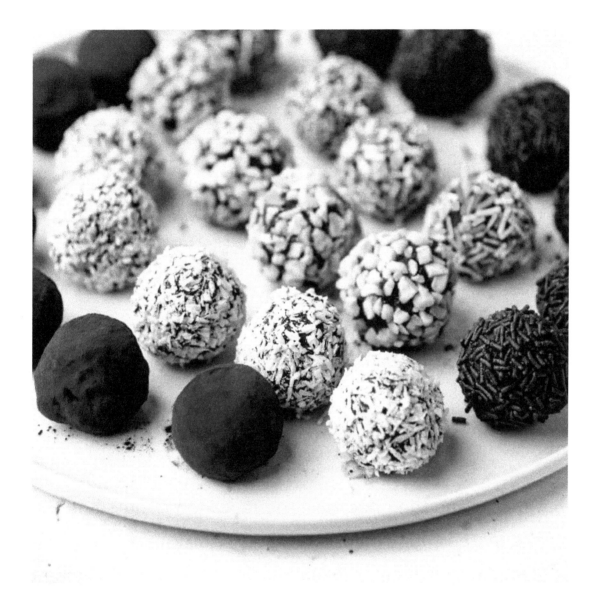

Preparation time: 5 minutes

Cooking time: 10 minutes

Servings: 10

Ingredients:

- 1 cup ghee, melted
- 3 tablespoons macadamia nuts, chopped
- ¼ cup stevia
- 5 tablespoons unsweetened coconut powder
- 2 tablespoons cocoa powder
- 1 cup water

Directions:

In a bowl, combine the ghee with the macadamia nuts and the rest of the ingredients except the water, whisk really well and shape medium balls out of this mix. Add the water to the instant pot, add the steamer basket, arrange the balls inside, put the lid on and cook on High for 10 minutes. Release the pressure fast for 5 minutes and serve the balls cold.

Nutrition: calories 200, fat 22.4, fiber 0.5, carbs 0.9, protein 0.5

Mint Cookies

Preparation time: 10 minutes

Cooking time: 15 minutes

Servings: 4

Ingredients:

- ¼ cup Erythritol

- ½ teaspoon dried mint

- ¼ teaspoon mint extract

- 4 teaspoons cocoa powder

- 2 egg whites

- ¼ teaspoon baking powder

- ¼ teaspoon lemon juice

- 1 cup water, for cooking

Directions:

Whisk the egg whites gently and add dried mint. Then add Erythritol, mint extract, cocoa powder, baking powder, and lemon juice. Stir the mass until smooth. Pour water in the instant pot. Line the instant pot trivet with the baking paper. Place it in the instant pot. With the help of the scooper make 4 cookies and put them on the trivet. Close the lid and cook the cookies on manual mode (high pressure) for 15 minutes. When the time is over, make a quick pressure release. Open the lid and transfer the cookies on the plate or chopping board. Cool the cookies well.

Nutrition: calories 13, fat 0.3, fiber 0.6, carbs 1.3, protein 2.1

Vanilla and Cocoa Cream

Preparation time: 5 minutes

Cooking time: 5 minutes

Servings: 4

Ingredients:

- 1 and ½ cups heavy cream

- 3 tablespoons swerve

- 2 tablespoons cocoa powder

- 1 teaspoon vanilla extract

- 1 and ½ cups water

Directions:

In a bowl, combine the heavy cream with the rest of the ingredients except the water, whisk well and divide into 4 ramekins. Put the water in the instant pot, add the steamer basket, put the ramekins inside, put the lid on and cook on High for 5 minutes. Release the pressure fast for 5 minutes and serve the cream cold.

Nutrition: calories 216, fat 22.6, fiber 0.8, carbs 3.3, protein 1.7

Coconut Clouds

Preparation time: 10 minutes

Cooking time: 6 minutes

Servings:2

Ingredients:

- •2 egg whites

- •4 tablespoons coconut flakes

- •1 tablespoon almond meal

- •¼ teaspoon ghee

- •1 teaspoon Erythritol

Directions:

Whisk the egg whites until strong peaks. Then slowly add the almond meal and coconut flakes. Add Erythritol and stir the mixture until homogenous with the help of the silicone spatula. Toss ghee in the instant pot and preheat it on sauté mode for 2 minutes. Then with the help of the spoon, make the clouds from egg white mixture and put them in the hot ghee. Close the lid and cook the dessert on sauté mode for 4 minutes.

Nutrition: calories 74, fat 5.4, fiber 1.3, carbs 2.4, protein 4.6

Plums Pie

Preparation time: 10 minutes

Cooking time: 30 minutes

Servings: 8

Ingredients:

For the crust:

- 1 cup coconut, unsweetened and shredded

- 1 cup pecans, chopped

- ¼ cup ghee, melted

For the filling:

- 8 ounces cream cheese

- 4 ounces strawberries

- 2 tablespoons water

- ½ tablespoon lime juice

- 1 teaspoon swerve

- ½ cup heavy cream

- 1 and ½ cups water

Directions:

In a bowl, combine the coconut with the pecans and the ghee, stir well and press on the bottom of a lined pie pan. In a second bowl, combine the cream cheese with the rest of the ingredients except the water, whisk well, pour over the crust and spread well. Add the water to the instant pot, add the steamer basket, put the pie pan inside, put the lid on and cook on High for 30 minutes. Release the pressure naturally for 10 minutes, cool the pie down, slice and serve.

Nutrition: calories 221, fat 22.4, fiber 1.2, carbs 3.6, protein 2.8

Shortbread Cookies

Preparation time: 15 minutes

Cooking time: 14 minutes

Servings: 6

Ingredients:

- 1 egg, beaten

- ¾ teaspoon salt

- 1 tablespoon almond butter

- 1 teaspoon coconut oil

- ¼ teaspoon baking powder

- ¼ teaspoon apple cider vinegar

- 1 tablespoon Erythritol

- 5 oz coconut flour

- 1 cup water, for cooking

Directions:

Mix up egg with salt, almond butter, coconut flour, and baking powder. Add apple cider vinegar, coconut oil, and Erythritol. Knead the dough and make 6 balls from it. Then press the balls gently with the help of the hand palm and place in the non-sticky instant pot baking tray. Pour water and insert the trivet in the instant pot. Place the tray with cookies on the trivet and close the lid. Cook the cookies on manual mode (high pressure) for 14 minutes. When the time is over, make a quick pressure release and open the lid. Transfer the cooked cookies on the plate and let them cool well.

Nutrition: calories 135, fat 5.5, fiber 10.4, carbs 17.5, protein 4.9

Vanilla Cream Mix

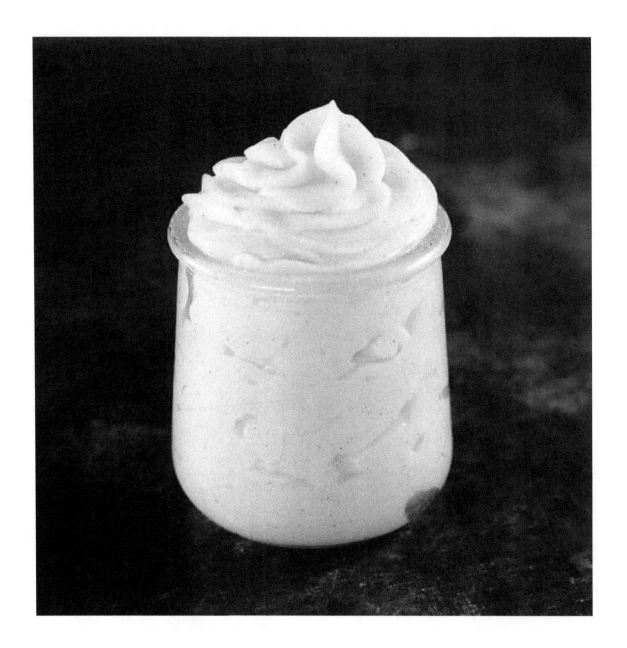

Preparation time: 10 minutes

Cooking time: 20 minutes

Servings: 4

Ingredients:

- 1 tablespoon vanilla extract

- 4 tablespoons butter

- 4 tablespoons sour cream

- 16 ounces cream cheese, soft

- ½ cup swerve

- ½ cup cocoa powder

- 1 cup heavy cream

- 2 cups water

Directions:

In a bowl, combine the vanilla with the butter and the rest of the ingredients except the water, whisk well and divide into 4 ramekins. Add the water to the instant pot, add the steamer basket, put the ramekins inside, put the lid on and cook on High for 20 minutes. Release the pressure naturally for 10 minutes, and serve the cream cold.

Nutrition: calories 330, fat 20.2, fiber 1.6, carbs 5.4, protein 5.8

Lime Bars

Preparation time: 20 minutes

Cooking time: 10 minutes

Servings: 6

Ingredients:

- ½ cup coconut flour

- 2 teaspoons coconut oil

- ¼ teaspoon baking powder

- ½ tablespoon cream cheese

- 1/3 cup coconut cream

- 2 tablespoons lime juice

- 1 teaspoon lime zest, grated

- 2 tablespoons Erythritol

•1 cup water, for cooking

Directions:

Knead the dough from coconut flour, coconut oil, baking powder, and cream cheese. When the mixture is soft and non-sticky, it is prepared. Then line the instant pot bowl with baking paper. Place the dough inside and flatten it in the shape of the pie crust (make the edges). Close the lid and cook it on sauté mode for 5 minutes. After this, switch off the instant pot. Make the filling: mix up coconut cream, lime juice, lime zest, and Erythritol. Then pour the liquid over the cooked pie crust and cook it on sauté mode for 5 minutes more. When the time is over, transfer the cooked meal in the freezer for 10 minutes. Cut the dessert into bars.

Nutrition: calories 88, fat 6, fiber 4.3, carbs 7.9, protein 1.7

Mascarpone Cheesecake

Preparation time: 5 minutes

Cooking time: 15 minutes

Servings: 6

Ingredients:

- 2 tablespoons butter, soft

- 1 cup heavy cream

- 2 ounces chocolate, melted

- ½ cup swerve

- 12 ounces mascarpone cheese

- 1 and ½ teaspoon cocoa powder

- 1 egg, whisked

- Cooking spray

- 1 cup water

Directions:

In a bowl, combine the butter with the cream and the rest of the ingredients except the cooking spray and the water and whisk well. Grease a cake pan with the cooking spray and pour the mix inside. Add the water to the instant pot, add the steamer basket, put the cake pan inside, put the lid on and cook on High for 15 minutes. Release the pressure fast for 5 minutes, cool the cheesecake down and serve.

Nutrition: calories 263, fat 22.2, fiber 0.3, carbs 6, protein 8.5

Cookies

Preparation time: 20 minutes

Cooking time: 5 minutes

Servings: 2

Ingredients:

- ¼ teaspoon peppermint extract

- 2 tablespoons almond flour

- 1 teaspoon heavy cream

- ½ teaspoon butter, softened

- ¼ oz dark chocolate

Directions:

Preheat the instant pot on sauté mode for 3 minutes. Then add almond flour, butter, and heavy cream. Add peppermint extract and dark chocolate. Saute the mixture for 2 minutes. Stir well. Then line the tray with baking paper. With the help of the spoon make the cookies from the peppermint mixture and transfer on the prepared baking paper. Refrigerate the cookies for 20 minutes.

Nutrition: calories 199, fat 17.1, fiber 3.3, carbs 8.1, protein 6.2

Creamy Chocolate Avocado Mix

Preparation time: 5 minutes

Cooking time: 5 minutes

Servings: 4

Ingredients:

- 2 avocados, peeled, pitted and chopped

- 1 cup heavy cream

- ½ cup chocolate chips

- ¼ cup swerve

- 1 teaspoon vanilla extract

- 1 cup water

Directions:

In your food processor, combine the avocados with the rest of the ingredients except the water, pulse well and divide into 4 ramekins. Put the water in the instant pot, add the steamer basket, put the ramekins inside, put the lid on and cook on High for 5 minutes. Release the pressure fast for 5 minutes, and serve the creamy mix really cold.

Nutrition: calories 283, fat 24.6, fiber 4, carbs 4.8, protein 2.8

Macadamia Cookies

Preparation time: 15 minutes

Cooking time: 13 minutes

Servings: 4

Ingredients:

- 1 oz macadamia nuts, chopped

- ½ cup coconut flour

- 2 tablespoons butter

- 1 tablespoon Erythritol

- 1 egg, beaten

- 2 tablespoons flax meal

- 1 cup water, for cooking

Directions:

In the mixing bowl mix up macadamia nuts, coconut flour, butter, Erythritol, egg, and flax meal. Knead the non-sticky dough. Then cut the dough into the pieces and make balls from them. Pour water and insert the trivet in the instant pot. Line the trivet with baking paper and put the dough balls on it. Cook the cookies for 13 minutes on manual mode (high pressure). When the time is over, make a quick pressure release and transfer the cookies on the plate.

Nutrition: calories 193, fat 15.5, fiber 6.6, carbs 10.1, protein 4.8

Vanilla Chocolate Cupcakes

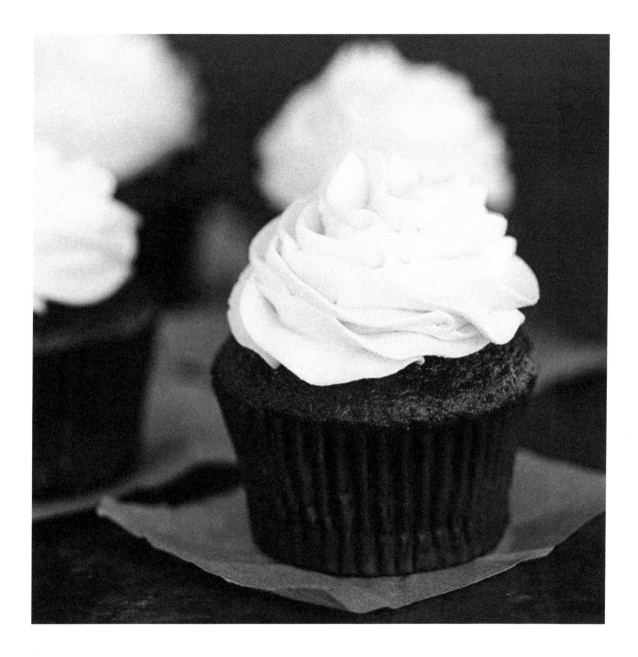

Preparation time: 10 minutes

Cooking time: 20 minutes

Servings: 12

Ingredients:

- ½ cup butter, melted

- ½ cup avocado oil

- ½ cup coconut, shredded

- 2 ounces chocolate, chopped

- ¼ cup cocoa powder

- ¼ teaspoon vanilla extract

- ¼ cup swerve

- 1 cup water

Directions:

In a bowl, combine the butter with the oil and the rest of the ingredients except the water and whisk really well. Line a cupcake pan that fits the instant pot with parchment paper and divide the chocolate mix inside. Put the water in the instant pot, add the steamer basket, add the cupcake pan inside, put the lid

110

on and cook on High for 20 minutes. Release the pressure naturally for 10 minutes and serve the cupcakes cold.

Nutrition: calories 243, fat 23.2, fiber 2.7, carbs 6.8, protein 2

Keto Pralines

Preparation time: 10 minutes

Cooking time: 8 minutes

Servings: 6

Ingredients:

- ½ cup butter

- 5 tablespoons heavy cream

- 2 tablespoons Erythritol

- ¼ teaspoon xanthan gum

- 4 pecans, chopped

Directions:

Place the butter in the instant pot and melt it on sauté mode. Add heavy cream and Erythritol. Stir the mixture well and sauté for 2 minutes. After this, add xanthan gum and pecan. Stir well and cook the mixture for 3 minutes more. Line the baking tray with baking paper. With the help of the spoon, place the pecan mixture in the tray in the shape of circles. Refrigerate the pralines until they are solid.

Nutrition: calories 254, fat 26.6, fiber 3.5, carbs 4.2, protein 1.4

Cream Cheese and Blackberries Mousse

Preparation time: 4 minutes

Cooking time: 4 minutes

Servings: 4

Ingredients:

- 8 ounces cream cheese

- 1 teaspoon serve

- 1 cup heavy cream

- 1 tablespoon blackberries

- 1 cup water

Directions:

In a bowl, mix the cream with the other ingredients except the water, whisk well and divide into 2 ramekins. Put the water in the instant pot, add the steamer basket, put the ramekins inside, put the lid on and cook on High for 4 minutes. Release the pressure fast for 4 minutes and serve the mousse really cold.

Nutrition: calories 202, fat 20.5, fiber 0.1, carbs 1.7, protein 3.3

Blueberry Crisp

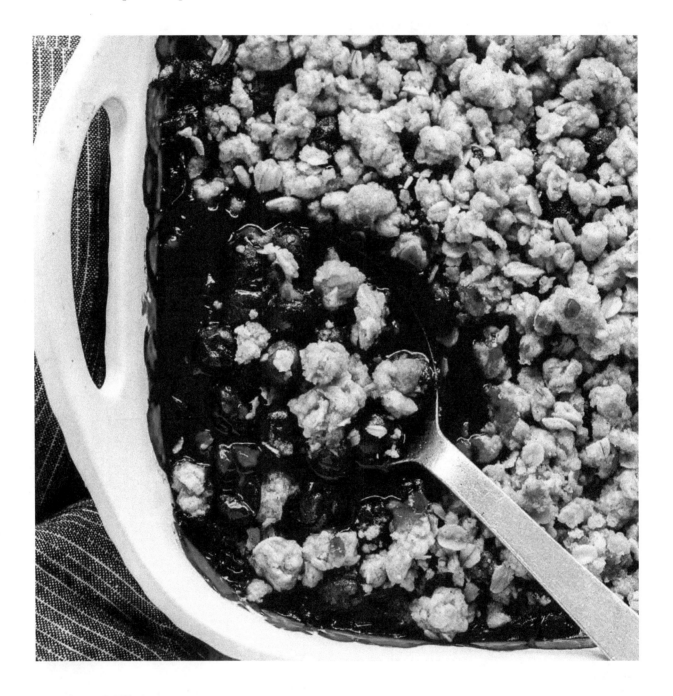

Preparation time: 10 minutes

Cooking time: 6 minutes

Servings: 4

Ingredients:

- ¼ cup almonds, blended

- 1 teaspoon butter

- 1 teaspoon flax meal

- 1 tablespoon Erythritol

- ½ cup cream cheese

- ½ cup blueberries

- 1 oz peanuts, chopped

Directions:

Toss butter in the instant pot and melt it on sauté mode. Add almonds and flax meal. Cook the mixture on sauté mode for 4 minutes. Stir it constantly. After this, cool the mixture well. Whisk the cream cheese with Erythritol. Then put ½ of cream cheese mixture in the serving glasses. Add ½ part of the almond mixture and ½ part of blueberries. Repeat the same steps with remaining mixtures. Top the dessert with chopped peanuts.

Nutrition: calories 197, fat 17.8, fiber 2, carbs 6, protein 5.6

Conclusion

The instantaneous pot is such an innovative as well as advanced cooking tool. It has gotten many followers around the world. The immediate pot allows you to prepare tasty meals for all your family in an issue of minutes as well as with minimal effort. The best feature of the immediate pot is that you do not require to be a specialist chef to make yummy cooking banquets. You simply require the best components as well as the right instructions. That's just how you'll get the most effective immediate pot dishes.

This great culinary overview you've simply uncovered is greater than an easy split second pot cooking journal. It is a Ketogenic instant pot recipes collection you will find extremely valuable. The Ketogenic diet will certainly offer you the energy boost you require, it will make you lose the extra weight and also it will certainly enhance your total health in an issue of days. This collection consists of the best Ketogenic instant pot meals you can prepare in the comfort of your own residence. All these meals are so flavored and distinctive and also they all taste extraordinary.

So, if you are following a Ketogenic diet plan and you own an instantaneous pot, get your own duplicate of this cookbook as well as start your Ketogenic cooking experience. Prepare the best Ketogenic instant pot meals and appreciate them all!

CPSIA information can be obtained
at www.ICGtesting.com
Printed in the USA
LVHW062016260521
688586LV00017B/634